The Beginner's Guide to Intermittent Fasting

Rapid Weight Loss, Building Lean Muscle and Fat Burning for People Who Hate Dieting

Introduction

I want to thank you and congratulate you for downloading the book, *"The Beginner's Guide to Intermittent Fasting: Rapid Weight Loss, Building Lean Muscle and Fat Burning for People Who Hate Dieting"*.

This book contains basic information about intermittent fasting as well as proven steps and strategies on how to practice it regularly.

Losing weight can be challenging, especially if you are not used to following a dietary plan that imposes restrictions on you, such as what you should and shouldn't eat. There is also the risk of you having chosen a diet that turns out to be too difficult or too tedious for you to follow over time. This can result in the exertion of immense effort in exchange for very little progress. Worse still, whatever progress you've made can be easily offset the moment you go back to your old eating habits, hence leaving you no better than when you started.

If you still want to lose weight or at least prevent more unwanted pounds from piling up, intermittent fasting is a way for you to achieve that without placing too much of a burden on you. Although it still requires you to eat less frequently than what you're used to as with other forms of fasting, it is easier to manage, it allows you to incorporate some variety in an otherwise repetitive eating plan, and it offers plenty of health benefits besides weight loss.

This is not some new weight loss craze. This is an actual eating plan that has been around even before any of us were born. In other words, it is so effective that it lasted long enough to be practiced ages after it first came into the picture. Why not give it a shot? Read this book and prepare to be amazed at how something as simple as fasting can make a big, positive impact in your life.

Thanks again for downloading this book, I hope you enjoy it!

Table of Contents

Chapter 1 – Intermittent Fasting Explained

So many weight loss plans promising positive results have come and gone over the years. Some advocate eating more of specific types of food (e.g. low carb, paleo), some suggest reducing one's overall intake of all foods or only a few specific types, some emphasize exercise rather than dieting, and there are even combinations of all three. The huge selection of such plans and what they promise can already make it difficult for anyone to decide which one to adopt and practice for the long term.

You've probably come to know about some of the different weight loss plans yourself but may be reluctant to try them out due to their complexity. Very few of the most worthwhile things in this world are easy to achieve, but that doesn't mean you will need to endure difficulty the whole time you are adhering to your chosen plan. The first step will always be the hardest as your body is still adjusting to this new way of doing things. After that, it gets easier and easier.

While there are many authors or so-called "gurus" that will tell you that their method is the ONLY WAY to effortless weight loss, I refuse this way of thinking. Many of the weight loss plans out there can work if done properly. I am a big believer in intermittent fasting as an efficient tool for your weight loss journey but am always open to learning many different paths that can be taken towards achieving your ideal body. The key is to pick one and start! As you have picked up this book, I hope that I can give you a glimpse into the world of intermittent fasting and how easy it can be to get started! Let's get into the nitty-gritty.

What is intermittent fasting?

Intermittent fasting is a simple strategy of ensuring weight loss by maintaining your overall caloric intake even though you are eating fewer meals on some days than you normally would.

If you assume that intermittent fasting can help you lose weight just like any other form of fasting (theoretically, at least), then you're right. However, it is not simply depriving yourself of the foods you want to eat. Depending on your chosen intermittent fasting method, you can still indulge into some of your favorite foods; the only catch is that you can't eat these or any other foods WHENEVER you want. You need to learn to eat just enough to make sure you have sufficient calories to last you through the day, and perhaps even into the day after.

Right now, you might be wondering why you still need to consume calories over time if your goal is to lose weight. "Won't consuming calories actually make me gain weight?" you might ask.

It is a common misconception that not consuming any calories automatically equates to weight loss. The truth is even the little things you do every day such as walking require calories. Remember that a calorie is a unit of measure of body heat energy. You will need to maintain a certain level of caloric intake every day even if you will be doing virtually nothing (though it is highly advised that you also incorporate some form of exercise in your weekly routine).

Intermittent fasting is not the same as dieting—it's actually a lot easier

Many people who want to lose weight by going on a diet often fall into the trap of giving up when things get tough or when they start to miss eating their favorite foods. The first few days might seem like a breeze, but when the feeling of despair or longing (for one's favorite food that is) sets in, it is easy to temporarily forget about what you are trying to achieve in the first place and resort to something easier or more appealing. With intermittent fasting, you can still eat some of your favorite foods. You just need to learn to eat at specific intervals instead of as often as you want.

Intermittent fasting is more about *when* you eat, not *what* you eat. It is not some weight loss gimmick that just came about recently only to be eventually dismissed as a fad. It is an effective eating plan that has been around for a long time, much longer than you may probably think.

How does intermittent fasting work?

When we eat, the food we have just consumed is processed by the body over the course of several hours, in effect burning the food to become the energy that we will need for the day. But what happens during times when you are unable to eat anything at all? Won't you starve to death? Will your body still have an available source of energy should you find yourself in such a situation? Fortunately, it is possible for the human body to last several hours, or even a whole day, without very little to no food.

People have always believed that eating a meal loaded with sugar or other carbohydrates was the only way for the body to have the energy it will need for even just a few hours. What many people do not know is that the body was designed to draw energy from other sources as well. It is just that the body is wired to burn carbohydrates before anything else because these are more readily available. One way of ensuring the use of non-carbohydrates as energy sources is fasting, which is basically a period of eating fewer meals than usual to enable the body to use its energy reserves. Unsurprisingly, the idea of eating fewer meals than what one is used to does not seem appealing. Many think that they would be depriving themselves of something that was so essential to living a full and satisfying life (i.e. food).

Yes, it can be done

Are you afraid of the idea of fasting? Or have you tried it once but then decided that not eating anything for even just a few hours will do you more harm than good? You may not have realized it, but you have been practicing one particular form of fasting your whole life: sleeping. You do not eat any food while you are sleeping, nor can you even think about eating while you are off in dreamland (probably except when you happen to dream about food). The point here is that you can easily go 7 to 8 hours straight without adding anything in your stomach and still wake up alive and in one piece, albeit a bit hungry.

Your body is able to last that long without any food thanks in part to the stores of glycogen in your liver and in your muscles. Glycogen is a type of starch that is produced when your body converts carbohydrates into energy. It consists of some of the excess carbohydrates that are not immediately consumed as fuel by your body and instead get stored for later use. Glycogen often gets nearly depleted after you have slept for 7 to 8 hours, hence making you feel hungry when you wake up. The term "breakfast" consequently came about because it refers to the meal you eat to break the lengthy fasting period you had the night before.

Let's say that you've just woken up from an 8-hour sleep and, as a result, your glycogen reserves are nearly empty. However, for some reason, you end up not eating anything for breakfast on that day. Will your body still have enough sources of energy to carry you through the next few hours? Indeed, it will.

After your body has converted carbohydrates from the food you eat into energy, some of the excess that does not end up as glycogen will instead be converted by the liver into fat which will then end up in various parts of your body. Unlike glycogen which ends up only in the liver and in some muscles, fat enjoys much greater storage space in your body in spite of it being more difficult to access than glycogen. Carbohydrates end up as fat elsewhere in the body simply because it can store only a relatively limited amount of glycogen.

However, like glycogen, fat can be converted into energy for the body. This happens when the nervous system triggers the adrenal glands to send the hormone norepinephrine to the fat cells so that they can be broken down into free fatty acids that are more easily burned for energy.

Fat burning will proceed uninterrupted only if you break your fast by eating a meal with a limited number of calories. This is because doing so ensures you do not consume a rather large excess of carbohydrates that will automatically be burned before the fat that has been made readily available. Eating a low-calorie meal to break the fast also activates the sympathetic nervous system which triggers the body's fight or flight response. As a result, you become fully alert and you don't feel the effects of hunger as much as if you ate a bigger meal at the end of your fast.

Otherwise, eating a big meal to break your fast will instead activate the parasympathetic nervous system which leads to the production of glycogen. Glycogen production and fat burning cannot happen at the same time, so the latter automatically ceases to make way for the former.

When you practice intermittent fasting, you are "teaching" your body to immediately burn any stored fats for energy by making these much easier to access than what is otherwise possible. If you have not eaten any food, your body will eventually operate on autopilot by prioritizing any readily available stored fats as its energy source. The body is considered to be in the "fasted state" when this happens. Fat burning leads to weight loss, which is the ultimate goal of this fasting method.

You get your body geared for the fasted state by fasting for the better part of a day over the course of a week or so. You can start by skipping breakfast for a few days and then you adopt the habit of eating at specific times. Going for long periods in between without eating anything, your body will learn to thrive while in the fasted state. You kick the habit of eating three big meals or even six small meals a day and instead learn to eat only no more than one light meal (or its total calorie equivalent in snacks) on some days.

If you've always thought that this is impossible, it might interest you to know that our prehistoric hunter-gatherer ancestors had no other choice. They had no way of telling when it was time for them to eat. They didn't even have the means to prepare equally portioned meals that would have enabled them to eat only what was necessary and then preserve the rest of their available food to be consumed later. They ate whatever was available at any given time, which often meant going for long periods without anything in their stomachs because food wasn't always available in the regions where they lived.

Despite all the limitations our ancestors faced, they were able to survive. Their bodies became strong and resilient enough to endure those same difficulties again and again in order to live. Our bodies are not really wired differently from how theirs were, so there is no reason for you to think we cannot live through a similar experience. In fact, some of the modern innovations available today can help you practice proper fasting with convenience that our ancestors could only dream about during their time.

The real challenge

Perhaps the first and biggest hurdle you need to overcome is getting your body to successfully adapt to your new routine. It's not easy to just switch to eating only one or even two full meals a day on certain days of the week if you've become used to eating three meals a day your whole life. Sure, it might be doable the first day, but you'll soon enough find yourself craving for something to eat during the period that you're supposed to be fasting. Before you know it, you're already munching on a cheeseburger and essentially ruining your plans even before you've made any real progress.

Don't worry for it is perfectly normal for you to feel hungry when you have not eaten anything for even just a few hours, whether or not you intentionally deprive yourself of food. If your daily routine is similar to others in terms of eating a full meal every three hours, your brain will be wired to "think" that this is the normal way of doing things. Your body thus becomes used to this pattern, and so it expects this pattern to occur at around the same times day after day. As a result, if it has been three hours following your last meal and you have not yet eaten anything since then, your body will start to get hungry because it *expects* to be fed at that particular time. It is this feeling of hunger that you need to overcome if you want to achieve positive results through intermittent fasting. Over time, your body will learn not to expect any food all day as the feeling of hunger will become less and less distracting every time you fast.

Again, if you want motivation and proof that it is possible, let's look at our cave-dwelling ancestors. They did not have the luxury of being able to eat three full meals at regular intervals within a 24-hour window. They ate whatever they could whenever they could, which often meant several hours elapsing between their meals. If our ancestors could successfully fast intermittently, SO CAN YOU!

Technology changed everything in the centuries that followed. We now enjoy breakthroughs such as cooked meals, proper portioning, and food storage. It therefore became possible for anyone to eat scheduled meals throughout the day for convenience's sake and to keep the rest of their food long enough for them to consume at a later time. As a result, the norm of being able to last several hours between meals became all but forgotten. Regardless of how meals you consume from morning to night, there is nothing inherently wrong with this setup. However, if you want your metabolism to be as efficient as possible to minimize the occurrence of unused energy in your body, you may need to start eating fewer meals on some days.

Intermittent fasting hopes to teach people the basic premise that eating what is necessary, ONLY WHEN IT IS NECESSARY, will still give the body the energy it needs as well as ensure weight loss.

How about if I simply eat a larger number of smaller-sized meals throughout the day?

It has been said that eating more frequently will burn more calories and thus lessen the occurrence of unused energy being stored as glycogen and fat in the body. This can be done by reducing the amount of food you eat for each of your meals. This approach seems to make some sense, but depends primarily on your calorie intake difference.

When you eat, the number of calories you burn is proportional to how big or how small your meal is. Let's say that, every day, you're used to eating three full meals that happen to have 600 calories each and then decide to switch to six smaller meals with only 300 calories each. In this case, the total calorie count for both meal plans is the same: 1800 calories. Thus, whether you eat three full meals or six smaller meals throughout the day, you are likely to end up consuming the same number of calories anyway. This is obviously not the solution if you're aiming for weight loss. With that said, if you can make do with lower overall calories for the six meals (e.g. 250 calories each which would result in 1500 calories total), you can see some progress.

The key is to modify your calorie intake, not the quantity/size of meals. As mentioned earlier, calorie calculators will give you an understanding of what your ideal calorie consumption per day should be in order to achieve your desired weight loss goals.

Is fasting the only thing I need to do?

Now you might be asking: can the body survive on its fat stores alone? It can't. Fat deposits are still liable to be fully depleted, and that's why you still need to eat just the right amount of carbohydrates at regular intervals to help stabilize your overall caloric intake. Carbohydrates can also benefit your health by regulating proper brain and body functioning, which is why you cannot just eliminate them from your diet completely. You can't have fat deposits unless you have consumed an excess of carbohydrates, as has already been explained in the preceding paragraphs.

Remember that this eating plan is a form of fasting; it is not the same as starving yourself by not eating anything at all. You still need to replenish your body with new calories much less frequently as opposed to every 3 to 4 hours as you used to do every day. The key is in finding the right balance between eating and allowing the body to use its available stored energy, the results of which are weight loss and more efficient conversion of food into energy.

Regardless of whatever weight loss program you will pick up, there are usually two factors that get discussed: diet and exercise. Since this book is on intermittent fasting, we focus on the diet aspect. I do want to mention though that I highly recommend incorporating some form of exercise as well!

Chapter 2 – Other Benefits of Intermittent Fasting

Weight loss isn't the only good thing that you can get from intermittent fasting. It's also not just your body that benefits from it either. Read on to know more about the positive changes that properly practiced intermittent fasting can bring into your life.

- It reduces the risk of insulin resistance and diabetes

  When your body has adjusted to the point that effective intermittent fasting is possible, it becomes more efficient in converting into energy any carbohydrates that you consume. This happens because of greater insulin sensitivity, and the result is less glucose circulating in the bloodstream over time. Glucose is derived from the carbohydrates you have consumed but have not been converted into glycogen and fat, both of which are stored in the body and may be used as fuel at a later time. With less glucose circulating in the bloodstream, there is less risk of the pancreas being unable to produce enough insulin. One result of this is that the body becomes resistant to the effects of this all-important hormone, which could lead to diabetes if not properly addressed.

- It helps in the fight against cancer

  Some studies have been conducted to determine whether or not intermittent fasting can help cancer patients in any way, and the results so far are promising. One study involving 10 patients showed that intermittent fasting done before chemotherapy resulted in diminished side effects of the treatment. Another study involving the alternate-day fasting method showed that fasting before chemotherapy improved cure rates as well as increased the likelihood of survival.

- It can also improve mental health

Intermittent fasting has been found to increase synaptic plasticity, which is a biological process that enhances the brain's ability to change and adapt to new information, hence improving learning and memory retention. It also leads to the growth of new neurons, which in turn lowers the risk of neurodegenerative diseases such as Alzheimer's and Parkinson's. Intermittent fasting can even help prevent anxiety and depression; even if these mood disorders have already set in, fasting can nonetheless have a therapeutic effect on them.

You're probably wondering how an eating plan that is touted as a big help in ensuring weight loss can also have positive effects on the brain. Deliberately depriving yourself of food from time to time actually challenges all your body systems, in effect making them stronger and more resilient over time. Think of it as giving your whole body a workout. After all, you can't have stronger muscles if you don't regularly push them to their limits.

- It can help in the body's development

Intermittent fasting has been found to boost levels of human growth hormone (HGH) by as much as five-fold. HGH is an essential component in activities including but not limited to cell repair and regeneration, calcium retention, protein synthesis, growth of internal organs other than the brain, and strengthening of the immune system. This has led many to tout this hormone as a modern-day fountain of youth.

- You end up spending less money

If you eat fewer meals than you used to eat every day, you don't have to cook as often as you used to, and that translates into a shorter list whenever you go shopping for groceries. You don't have to do the dishes as often, either, and that translates into additional savings for you. With intermittent fasting, not only will you lose weight, you may also have more money in the bank at the end of the day.

Chapter 3 – Drawbacks of Intermittent Fasting

As good as intermittent fasting is, there are some disadvantages that are backed by both science and the actual experiences of some of the people who have tried it. This, however, should not deter those who really want to try intermittent fasting for the right reasons. The key here is to keep track of your health at all times so that you fully reap the benefits of this proven method of regulating your body's caloric intake without putting yourself at unnecessary risk.

Here are some reasons intermittent fasting is not as easy to execute as many would hope.

- First of all, it's not for everyone

  If you suffer from diabetes, hypoglycemia, or any other health condition that has something to do with your body's blood sugar, intermittent fasting can be much more complex or not practical at all. If you still aim for weight loss but your condition requires you to stick to a normal eating pattern of at least three full meals a day, then intermittent fasting is obviously not the solution you need.

  Pregnant women are also discouraged from practicing intermittent fasting as the fetus in the womb will need a continuous supply of nutrients which can only be derived from the food that the mother regularly eats.

- It can become too easy for you to give up just as you're getting started

  Because you will be consuming less food while you're fasting, you could end up with fatigue, dizziness, difficulty in concentrating, and low energy during the first few days. All these things coming together could easily break your resolve to continue with the program despite the benefits. However, as long as you practice proper fasting, you will realize that you are not really depriving yourself and that your body is simply adjusting to what you want it to do.

- It could lead to increased cortisol levels

Cortisol is a stress hormone that is produced by the adrenal glands. Reduced food intake can lead to stress, especially among those who are fasting for the first time, as the body is not used to eating food less frequently than usual. The adrenal glands then release cortisol as a response. Some studies have found that there can be an increase in risk of anxiety due to elevated cortisol levels.

You can avoid stress and increased cortisol levels by not forcing yourself into your new routine. As will be explained in the succeeding chapters of this book, you will only truly reap the benefits of your chosen fasting method if it is something you can practice for the long term. Thus, if you find yourself constantly being stressed out just when you're starting out with a specific fasting method, you might need to try a different fasting method instead.

- It can lead to hormonal imbalance, especially in women

This will be explained in a later chapter.

In any case, it pays to be fully informed about intermittent fasting, and that includes its bad side as well. As mentioned earlier, I am not suggesting that intermittent fasting is the only solution to weight loss as it may not be for everyone. I want to be 100% transparent about the benefits and the drawbacks to give you a big picture summary of intermittent fasting. This list is not meant to discourage you from getting started on this plan if you feel you can benefit from it. This merely serves as a reminder of what you could expect whether you're just starting out with fasting or already farther along into your routine.

Chapter 4 – 7 Popular Intermittent Fasting Methods

One of the amazing things about intermittent fasting is that you are not limited to following just one specific method towards achieving your goals of more efficient energy burning and weight loss. You are free to choose from a variety of methods depending on your schedule, your usual diet, and various other factors. I highly recommend that you first consult with your doctor/nutritionist before starting any of these methods to ensure that they are done safely.

This chapter discusses some of the most popular intermittent fasting methods that are being practiced today as well as their respective advantages and disadvantages. The methods are listed here in no particular order.

1. Alternate-Day Fasting

The name of this fasting method already states what it will entail. In this method, you eat very little on one day, typically no more than a light meal (less than 500 calories for men and less than 400 for women), and then you eat as you normally would the following day. On the third day, you again limit yourself to only one meal and then eat whatever you like the day after. You simply keep this pattern up until you have achieved your intended weight loss then gradually switch to a slightly less restricting routine to maintain your target weight.

The proponents of this intermittent fasting method believe that through this, you will be consuming fewer calories than you normally would. And because you are consuming fewer calories overall, it is inevitable for you to lose weight over time.

Pros

- This fasting method focuses on restricting one's eating in order to help them lose weight. If you're not much into exercise, this could be a viable option for you. Some people who have tried this method reported losing up to two and a half pounds a week after simply having cut their calorie intake by as much as 20%.
- You can restrict calorie counting only to your fasting days, thus making this fasting method more manageable for people who have not tried any weight loss methods before.
- Since you will be fasting only every other day, you won't feel hungry every day, thereby lessening the risk that you would end up craving for something to eat and possibly ruining whatever progress you've already made. Limiting the periods wherein you will feel hungry to just every other day will make it easier for you to control yourself and thus eat no more than what you should on both fasting and non-fasting days. You can even schedule social occasions such as weekend barbecues on your non-fasting days and eat normally without fear of ruining your progress since you will be once again restricting your calorie intake the next day.
- One study conducted on overweight people revealed that the alternate-day fasting method was also effective in ensuring heart health as it helped lower cholesterol and blood pressure.

Cons

- Significantly cutting calorie intake on fasting days can make the feeling of hunger so overwhelming that it can easily discourage anyone who has just started practicing this fasting method. This is especially true among those who are trying a weight loss routine for the first time.
- It is possible you could also experience headaches and/or difficulty sleeping during your first couple of weeks on this fasting method.

- Consuming less than 500 calories on your fasting days can easily lead to depleted energy levels. People who wish to practice this method to achieve weight loss and lean muscle are thus discouraged from performing strenuous exercise during fasting days.
- Being allowed to eat normally on non-fasting days following the severe calorie restriction on fasting days can easily increase one's propensity to binge on non-fasting days. For example, if you're used to eating 2,000 total calories in one day and you eat only 500 calories on your fasting day, chances are you would consume nearly twice your normal daily calorie intake on your next fasting day. This will fully offset your calorie deficit, leaving you back at square one despite your initial efforts.

2. The 16/8 Method or "Lean Gains" Method

The 16/8 Method of intermittent fasting is also known as the Lean gains method. The approach to the 16/8 Method is trickier than that of the Alternate-Day Fasting method in that you do not simply limit yourself to just one light meal every other day. The "16/8" label came from the premise that a person needed to fast for 16 hours straight (14 hours for women) in any given 24-hour period and eat for the remaining 8 hours (10 hours for women) of that period, also known as a feeding window.

It doesn't matter whether you begin your 24 hours with the 16-hour fast or the 8-hour feeding window for as long as the 16-hour fast is done without any breaks in between. For example, you can't set your day up by having a 4-hour fast, a 4-hour feeding window, another 4-hour fast, another 4-hour feeding window, and then 8 hours of uninterrupted sleep in that order. You need to have a lengthy fasting period to give your body enough time to burn enough of your glycogen and fat reserves to ensure weight loss. You will never accomplish this if you stop even for a quick bite every 4 hours as you will be stuffing your body with more new carbohydrates to burn, hence leaving your glycogen and fat untouched for an indefinite period.

Pros

- One good thing about this diet is that you can easily incorporate one thing you do every day to help you get through the 16-hour window without any food: sleep. If you sleep for 8 hours within a 24-hour period, you would have already lasted 8 hours without eating, leaving you only 8 hours more to endure. Furthermore, you could easily adjust your sleep-fasting mix for as long as you get at least 8 hours of uninterrupted snooze time. For example, you could fast for 4 hours at 6:00PM on Monday, sleep for 8 hours beginning at 10:00PM, wake up at 6:00AM on Tuesday, and use the remaining 4 hours of the 16-hour window to fast. In this manner, you can limit the time you spend fasting after you sleep and before you have your next meal, thereby leaving you little time to feel the onset of hunger.
- The basic premise of the 16/8 Method never said anything about eating only a specific number of calories or having a fixed number of meals within the 8-hour feeding window. You are free to choose how to go about this step. Many of those who practice this method prepare three light meals which they can eat at regular intervals within the 8-hour feeding window. This is actually doable since our bodies have grown accustomed to eating three meals a day anyway.
- Unlike in the alternate-day fasting method, the body's energy reserves are not severely depleted during the fasting window under the 16/8 Method, allowing for workout periods to be squeezed in during fasting windows. This makes the method ideal for those who want to build muscle as well as lose weight.

Cons

- The 16/8 Method is somewhat limiting with regards to what a person can eat during the feeding window, especially if that person is aiming for building lean muscle as well. Although you are allowed to add variety to your daily meals, it doesn't necessarily mean you can eat anything you want. That means it's time to say goodbye to potato chips, cheeseburgers, doughnuts, and all the other junk you've been stuffing yourself with on a regular basis. If your normal routine also includes eating such foods, adjusting to this method will be more difficult.
- This fasting method was originally designed for bodybuilders. Hence, you will truly enjoy the benefits offered by this method only if you also practice a regular weight training protocol that also includes workout days and rest days in between.
- Beginners to this method are likely to experience mood swings for the first few days due to hunger felt during the fasting windows.

3. The 5:2 Diet

The 5:2 Diet is named such because it requires you to schedule a 7-day week in such a way that you have 5 days when you eat normally and 2 days when you limit yourself to no more than 600 total calories every day. Think of it as a variation of the alternate-day fasting method but without you having to fast every other day.

Pros

- You are free to choose when your normal eating days and when your fasting days will be for the week. Fasting days need not be consecutive, either. For example, you can eat normally from Monday to Wednesday, fast on Thursday, eat normally again on Friday and Saturday, and then devote your entire Sunday to fasting.

- For your fasting days, you are not limited to having only one low-calorie meal at a specific time of day. You can split these up into breakfast, lunch, and dinner for as long as your total calorie intake for the day does not exceed 600.
- The flexibility also means you are allowed to decide how long each of the gaps between meals will be during your fasting days. You could have shorter fasts instead of just one long fast that will last nearly the whole day. Shorter fasts are allowed since they give your digestive system a rest.

Cons
- Like the 16/8 Method, the 5:2 Diet is restrictive in terms of the food you can eat, even during the normal eating days. In other words, if your idea of "normal eating" also includes foods containing unhealthy sugars and fats, you should start ditching them in favor of healthier alternatives.
- As with the alternate-day fasting method, you could be compelled to binge following each fasting day to compensate after having "deprived" yourself.
- A study published in the New England Journal of Medicine in 2011 revealed that practicing the 5:2 Diet led to a reduction of some of the hunger-removing hormones found in the blood as well as an increase in hunger-causing hormones.

4. Eat Stop Eat

The Eat Stop Eat intermittent fasting method is even more restricting than the 5:2 diet in terms of how often you eat, though this in itself is not considered a disadvantage. This fasting method requires one or two 24-hour fasts per week, and in each 24-hour fast, you cannot consume any solid foods. However, you may drink water and low-calorie flavored beverages (the latter only in moderation) during your fasting periods.

The fundamental idea behind Eat Stop Eat is reduction of one's overall calorie intake by limiting meal frequency. The 24-hour fasts can induce a higher rate of fat-burning because the body does not have any new carbohydrates that it can burn for energy. It instead goes directly for the fat reserves.

Pros

- This intermittent fasting method is something that anyone can practice for the long term, whether or not they're bodybuilders.
- The program does not require you to go all-or-nothing at first. If you feel you cannot go 24 hours straight without eating anything, you can instead start by going for as long as possible without food. You can then gradually increase your fasting hours per fasting day until you are able to go the full stretch without anything in your stomach. To help you further in this, you can schedule your fast days during the days of the week when you'll be too busy or preoccupied to think about eating.
- The program does not forbid you to eat the foods you love, which means you have a better chance of not being overcome by sudden cravings on your fasting days.

Cons

- Some who have tried the Eat Stop Eat method reported that going 24 hours straight without any food can cause fatigue, headaches, mild anxiety, and irritability.
- Although sweetened low-calorie beverages may be consumed during fasting days (if you're grow tired of just water and want something else), the taste may trigger cravings for unhealthy sweets that you could result in binge eating.
- As mentioned earlier, the Eat Stop Eat program does not prohibit you from eating your favorite foods on your non-fasting days, but that is simply because it does not come with specific recommendations on what

you should eat. If you don't exercise proper discretion, you are liable to include foods that will do your health more harm than good.

5. The Warrior Diet or "One Meal a Day Diet"

The Warrior Diet intermittent fasting method promotes the concept of fasting for 20 hours and then eating a large meal afterwards, hence its alternate name of the "one meal a day diet." Although this method gives no specifics as to when you should fast and when you should eat, it is highly recommended that you start the 20-hour fasting phase when you go to sleep so that you will already cover 8 hours (just like in the 16/8 Method), fast for the next 12 hours after you wake up the following morning, and then have a 4-hour "overeating phase" at night. The nighttime meal helps the body recuperate since the nutrients from food that has just been consumed may be used for muscle repair and growth. Also, eating at night helps induce the body's production of hormones.

The first chapter of this book already mentioned the parasympathetic nervous system, particularly its role in the production of glycogen. This same system is especially active at night, and it becomes even more efficient after you have eaten a meal. Specifically, this system slows the heart rate, triggers intestinal function, and causes the muscles in the gastrointestinal tract to relax, promoting overall relaxation and digestion, hence this system's also being known as the "rest and digest system." Have you ever noticed that you sometimes feel sleepy after you have eaten a heavy meal regardless of the time of day? That's the parasympathetic nervous system at work.

The 4-hour overeating phase leaves little room for you to have two or more meals before your next 20-hour fasting period, so it's necessary to cram what you're going to eat during this phase into just one large meal.

Pros

- Being limited to just one full meal a day can actually be advantageous for you. By not having to make any meal planning, calorie counting, or other complex, distracting changes in your daily routine, you keep things simple and manageable, allowing you to focus on adjusting to your new eating schedule despite the temptation to go back to eating "normally" every day.
- You're allowed to eat a few light snacks throughout the 20-hour fast, thereby helping you easily curb any feelings of hunger in the hours before the overeating phase.
- Having your meals only at night is highly recommended because of the many benefits, but there's really no rule prohibiting you from having your big meal at any other time of the day. For example, if you have a weekend barbecue with your neighbors coming up, you can have your big meal of the day during the barbecue and then fast for the rest of the day until bedtime.

Cons

- This eating plan is rather restrictive in that it sets guidelines on what you should eat for your overeating phase meal and for any light snacks during the 20-hour fast. Specifically, it recommends that you start with vegetables, fruits, proteins, and fat and then eat carbohydrates last and only if you are still hungry. Although this approach can help trigger fat burning, which is the goal you wish to achieve through intermittent fasting, such a restriction can be difficult to adopt as a long-term practice as it gives you little room for variety. You could easily grow tired of this seemingly inflexible routine unless you are really committed to your goal.
- The overeating phase is named such simply because you will be eating a bigger than normal meal during this period. It does not mean you are to actually overeat through bingeing after your 20-hour fast.

Unfortunately, it can become challenging for those who are prone to bingeing to exercise self-control and to eat only the minimum allowable amount. This is especially true after one has fasted for most of the day.

6. Fat Loss Forever

The Fat Loss Forever intermittent fasting method combines the best parts of the 16/8 Method, Eat Stop Eat, and the Warrior Diet into one plan. It is a 7-day eating plan that begins with a cheat day immediately followed by a fasting period of a day and a half. For the remaining four and a half days, you incorporate the three aforementioned methods in any order. For example, if your cheat day is Monday and your 36-hour fast ends at noon on Wednesday, you can practice the 16/8 Method beginning on Wednesday afternoon (an 8-hour feeding window followed by a 16-hour fast), practice Eat Stop Eat from Thursday afternoon to Sunday, and then have a big meal on Sunday night (since the second fasting day of Eat Stop Eat and the 20-hour fast of the Warrior Diet will overlap on Sunday). There are way too many variations of this method to list in this introductory book of Intermittent Fasting. I recommend performing a simple Google search to help you find the many schedules, workouts and diet plans that could be used to practice this method. You can also check out the creator of this method: John Romaniello at omegabodyblueprint.com.

Pros
- This intermittent fasting method was devised as a solution to prevent fasting being done haphazardly. With everything following a specific schedule, you will learn to make a habit out of following different eating and fasting phases on different days to get the most out of the program.
- You get a full cheat day wherein you can eat anything you want—no restrictions whatsoever.

Cons

- Following the program can be confusing given the specific steps and the fact that no single fasting method is to be practiced all throughout. To remedy this, though, the program comes with a calendar that you can access online to guide you through each of the 7 days in a given cycle.
- The program includes a weight training regimen because of the inclusion of the 16/8 Method, so unless you regularly engage in muscle building workouts, this program might be difficult for you to follow.

7. Spontaneous Meal Skipping

This last method is not so much an actual eating plan as it is a way of getting beginners used to the practice of fasting. As such, it doesn't place any real restrictions on you other than to just skip a meal whenever it's time for you to eat but you're not hungry. You don't even need to schedule specific days of the week for fasting, nor do you have to perform any meal planning in advance. It's spontaneous because you can just choose to forego a certain meal when the time for eating that meal comes.

Pros

- Because Spontaneous Meal Skipping imposes very few restrictions, it can serve as a way for you to experiment with fasting to see whether or not you can practice it regularly by following a specific schedule.
- This plan doesn't explicitly state that you should eat or avoid specific foods. However, eating healthier meals every day will help you adjust more easily by giving you fewer carbohydrates to burn even if you follow your normal routine of having three full meals a day.

Cons

- The lack of structure will make it difficult for you to make a habit out of regular fasting. You basically choose not to eat at random times or because it is convenient for you to do so. Spontaneous Meal Skipping may serve as an effective dry run for you, but you cannot achieve any long-term positive results from fasting unless you adopt an eating plan that compels you to discipline yourself and to exercise self-control (i.e. learning not to eat even when you're hungry).

- This method can help you become familiar with how fasting is done as well as what it will require from you. However, it has a slim chance of yielding even just minimal weight loss because the practice of fasting is not done consistently.

Chapter 5 – Intermittent Fasting for Women

Given that the male and female human anatomies are different, intermittent fasting can also have different effects on men and women, which is not really surprising. What is alarming, though, is the fact that there are varying degrees of effectiveness that intermittent fasting has had on women who have tried it. Some women have reported positive results while others experienced more adverse effects on their health such as hormonal imbalance, metabolic disruption, and fertility issues. What's worse is that there is presently very little conclusive scientific literature explaining why intermittent fasting has such adverse effects on some of the women who have tried it, leading many to fast at their own risk if they really want to take this route.

All about the hormones

Hormonal imbalance seems to be the most notable among the known adverse effects that intermittent fasting has on women, though some health care and fitness experts argue that improper execution of one's chosen fasting method is the real culprit.

Reduced carbohydrate intake has a direct effect on the hunger hormones leptin and ghrelin. Specifically, reduced carbohydrate intake causes the body to sense that it is being starved, which then leads women to feel insatiable hunger. The hunger is actually the result of increased production of leptin and ghrelin, which is also the female body's automatic response if it senses the fetus in the womb is not getting enough of the nutrients it needs. This occurrence is true even among women who aren't pregnant simply because those two hormones are still present in their bodies. When the production of both these hormones ramps up, the result is hormonal imbalance. So much so that even the hormones that regulate key female reproductive functions such as ovulation are adversely affected.

What then follows is a period of binge eating after the fast to curb the feeling of hunger. After the bingeing, comes another lengthy period of fasting, only to be followed again by bingeing because the feeling of hunger once again becomes too much to bear. And the cycle goes on and the imbalance of hormones becomes much worse than before.

An alternative solution for women

If you're a woman and you want to practice intermittent fasting but without putting your hormones out of balance, you can first try to get a feel of what this type of fasting will require from you as well as how your body will react to the change in your routine. You can choose to devote no more than a whole day—preferably one when you are not particularly busy keeping to your other commitments so as to maintain your focus—to this "trial fast." This fast can last a full 24 hours, but you can opt to have a shorter fasting period depending on your level of confidence. You can also choose the start and end time as you see fit. Whichever way you go about it, you should not eat anything except only at the start and end times of your fast.

However long your fasting period will be, there should always be an allotted time in which you engage in something relaxing. This is partly to keep yourself too preoccupied to think of how hungry you are or how much time you have left before your next meal. You can do yoga, have your nails done, tend to your garden, or even take a nap—anything to keep your mind off the fact that you have not eaten anything at a time of day when you normally eat.

If your body responded well to the trial fast, that is if you do not feel any adverse effects and if you feel fasting is something you can sustain for the long term, you can then move on to performing your chosen fasting duration more regularly. You can go on a fast for one day every month, or even every week if you feel you're up to it. This is to slowly ease you into your new routine. Once you have no trouble performing monthly or weekly fasting, you can move on to what has been termed as Crescendo Fasting, which is a form of intermittent fasting done for only a few days a week instead of every day. This is easier to follow regularly as opposed to daily fasting that requires a lot more focus.

Crescendo Fasting requires you to fast on 2 to 3 nonconsecutive days per week. For example, you fast only on Mondays, Wednesdays, and Saturdays. This is to prevent your body from being overwhelmed by long periods without food even if you feel you have already mastered periodic fasting. You then complement your fast with gentle exercises like yoga or light cardio workouts on your fasting days and more intense activities such as strength training on your non-fasting days.

If done properly, Crescendo Fasting will help you achieve weight loss and leaner muscle without throwing your hormones out of balance. In any case, you should first consult your doctor to determine whether or not you should perform any fasting at all.

Chapter 6 – Foods to Eat and Foods to Avoid While Practicing Intermittent Fasting

There is no universal rule as to the foods you should eat and the foods you should avoid while you are on intermittent fasting. After all, the different intermittent fasting methods are varied with regards to their recommended and prohibited foods. Some are not very clear in that aspect, leading people who are fasting to use their own discretion in planning their meals for their eating periods.

This chapter will help you narrow down your choices if you're having trouble deciding what to include in your intermittent fasting regimen.

Foods to eat

- Proteins

  Eating meals rich in protein can help make you feel full longer as well as help build muscle. However, there are some high-protein foods that are also high in carbohydrates and therefore might not make ideal table fare for both fasting and non-fasting days.

  Some high-protein foods that you can consume while practicing intermittent fasting are listed below.

  - Meat and poultry – preferably of grass-fed animals
  - Fish
  - Eggs
  - Cottage cheese
  - Chia seeds
  - Lentils

    o Quinoa
    o Chickpeas

- Vegetables

Did you know that eating low-calorie vegetables can also make you feel full? Nearly all types of vegetables are low in calories while having more of the nutrients the body needs. This is especially true for leafy green vegetables.

You can have some variety when preparing meals and snacks with vegetables; you can steam them, stir-fry them with some spices for flavor, or just eat them raw in salad. You can even carry some sliced vegetables with you as snacks while you are on the go.

- Fat

Although fat is already high in calories, you still need to eat fatty foods to build up your body's fat stores that can serve as your energy source during your fasting periods.

Below are examples of foods that contain healthy fats.

    o Avocados
    o Dark chocolate
    o Nuts
    o Olive oil
    o Organic coconut oil
    o Grass-fed unsalted butter

- Carbohydrates

Now you may be thinking why carbohydrates are included in this list after what was discussed in the earlier chapters of this book. This is because carbohydrates nonetheless serve a number of important roles that include ensuring proper brain and body function. While you are practicing intermittent fasting, you are allowed to eat carbohydrate-laden foods but only in limited amounts, especially on your fasting days (depending on your chosen protocol). Ideally, you should eat no more than 100 grams of carbohydrates in every meal.

If you will incorporate bodybuilding in your intermittent fasting schedule, it is highly recommended that you eat carb-rich foods after a workout as carbohydrates are important for muscle development.

Below is a list of foods that are ideal sources of carbohydrates. Not only are they low in carbohydrates, they offer other health benefits as well.

- Barley – high in protein
- Black beans – source of protein and antioxidants
- Pumpkin seeds – source of zinc
- Walnuts – contains omega-3 fatty acids
- Breads and pastries made from almond flour – contains protein, antioxidants, and monounsaturated fat
- Fruits – Fruits are normally prohibited during intermittent fasting because of their high carbohydrate content. Specifically, many fruits are rich in fructose, a sugar that cannot be used by the body as energy. An excess of fructose can damage the liver and lead to insulin resistance among other things. However, if you want to include fruits in your daily meals, you may choose those with a low glycemic index (ideally 55 or below) as these have minimal impact on your blood sugar.

The following is a list of fruits with low glycemic index.

- Apples

- Cherries
- Grapefruit
- Grapes
- Oranges
- Peaches
- Pears
- Strawberries

Foods to avoid

- Sugar

  Sugary foods are the ones you should avoid the most while you are practicing intermittent fasting regularly. These foods are so high in carbohydrates that consuming them regularly will lead to an almost unending influx of carbohydrates into your body. The body will keep on burning carbohydrates for energy, in effect leaving your fat stores virtually untouched. Your body should become accustomed to burning fat for energy during your fasting periods, which is possible only if you limit your intake of sugary foods.

  Some intermittent fasting methods allow you to drink low-calorie sodas to help you curb any feelings of hunger during your fasting periods. However, their taste might end up triggering your cravings for sugary foods, putting you at risk of consuming more calories than necessary in your succeeding meals. You should instead strive to limit your beverage choices to water, coffee, and tea, which are not only low in carbohydrates but also provide you with a whole host of other health benefits.

  Some common sugary foods are in the list below. If you cannot avoid these foods entirely, you should gradually limit your intake of these to once or twice per week and incorporate healthier substitutes (some of which were discussed in the preceding chapter) in all your other meals.

- o Bread
- o Cake
- o Candy
- o Chocolate
- o Cold cereal
- o Cookies
- o Doughnuts
- o Energy bars
- o Honey
- o Ice cream
- o Jam
- o Juice
- o Milk
- o Muffins
- o Pancakes
- o Pasta
- o Pastries
- o Popcorn
- o Rice
- o Soda
- o Sports drinks

- Processed foods

Processed foods are known for their convenience, particularly in how they provide readily available meals and snacks for people who do not have time to prepare their own. They are also known for being able to be kept for long periods without spoiling. However, whatever benefits that can be gleaned from these foods are overshadowed by the low-quality proteins, added sugars, excess sodium, artificial fats, and added preservatives (which prolong their shelf life) that they contain. As such, these foods should not be included in your eating plan.

Those who wish to practice intermittent fasting are also advised to avoid processed foods that have the words "natural" and "organic" printed on their packaging. Such labels on the packages are not absolute guarantees that the foods they contain are indeed free of artificial additives with zero nutritional value.

Some processed foods that are to be avoided are listed below.

- o Bacon
- o Hamburgers
- o Hot dogs
- o Canned fruits and vegetables
- o Instant ramen
- o Ketchup
- o Margarine
- o Microwavable dinners

Chapter 7 – Some Tips and Tricks

Intermittent fasting presents a whole host of challenges even for people who are no strangers to dietary weight loss routines. The good news is that this eating plan was never designed to punish anyone by giving them instructions that are impossible to follow. In fact, there's no harm in making the journey a little easier for yourself for as long as you follow the basics.

Here are some tips that can help you if you're having trouble getting started or maintaining your momentum.

- Seek advice from a doctor before anything else

  Even if you know what it's like to follow a strict dietary plan or you feel you are confident enough to know how your body works, you cannot be 100% sure that you can practice intermittent fasting effectively just by following the steps you've read in a book or article. Your doctor can help you identify any issues about your health that you might have overlooked as some forms of fasting may aggravate certain health conditions that can adversely affect your body's blood-sugar retention.

- Get started through occasional fasting

  The steps involved in proper intermittent fasting regardless of method can be overwhelming for some. If you want to try intermittent fasting but feel that it involves a lot of work, you can gradually ease yourself into your new routine by skipping meals when it's convenient for you to do so. For example, on some days that you have a ton of work at the office, you can simply skip lunch and get cracking on all those reports, projects, and memos. Before you know it, you've accomplished a lot without ever having to grab a bite the whole day. You can easily compensate with a light meal as soon as you get home or just before you go to sleep.

- Always stay hydrated

Intermittent fasting gives the body an opportunity to detoxify by allowing the liver to process any toxins. These toxins can be easily excreted through urination or perspiration. Without any water intake, your body will be forced to rely on any water stored within to flush these toxins out. Detoxification can also be done in this manner, but because the body's stored water becomes depleted in the process, this will lead to dehydration. When you're dehydrated, you could suffer from decreased mental focus as well as greater susceptibility to fatigue. These two are the last things you would want to happen while you're doing your best to adapt to a new way of eating so that it becomes a habit for you.

To avoid this, always make sure to drink water at regular intervals throughout your fast. Don't limit yourself to the "5 to 8 glasses a day" rule that you learned in your elementary science classes. You will actually need to drink more during those days that you will be eating less food so as to prevent your body's water reserves from being depleted. Also remember not to gulp down a large volume of water all at once; otherwise you'll end up flushing it all out the next time you urinate, which will defeat the purpose of staying hydrated throughout your fast.

Some intermittent fasting methods, especially the 16/8 method, allow you to drink coffee during fasting periods if you want some variety or if you've already grown tired of the bland taste of water. This is acceptable for as long as you drink coffee in moderation. This is because the caffeine found in coffee is a diuretic, which means it can trigger increased production of urine. Urinating more frequently can cause you to quickly become dehydrated, so remember to limit your coffee intake and instead drink more water during your fasting periods.

- Keep yourself busy

If you're having trouble fasting because you can't stop thinking about how hungry you are, there are ways of addressing this without having to stop for a quick bite. One good thing about intermittent fasting is that it allows you to time your fasting periods as you see fit. For example, your fasting period can last for the whole time you are at the office or, during weekends, the hours you devote to exercise or quality time by yourself or with others. When you're focused on doing something productive, it becomes easier for you not to think about food until your next scheduled meal.

One way of keeping yourself busy is by exercise. Any glycogen in your liver can be further depleted since you'll be using it as energy during your workout. Further depletion of glycogen can increase insulin sensitivity, which can then lead to the food you eat being more efficiently converted into energy. This way, you not only lose weight, but you can build muscle as well.

- Have the right state of mind

It was discussed earlier in this book that even the simple act of getting started on intermittent fasting could make anyone susceptible to handicaps such as fatigue and lack of mental focus. It then becomes easy for anyone to give up right at the beginning before any real progress could be made. The key to overcoming this is continually having a positive attitude and your end goal in mind. For example, if you find yourself hungry and craving for something to eat with your next meal still hours away, you could simply tell yourself "At least I am slowly burning fat every day this way."

It doesn't matter how you motivate yourself to keep striving for the results you want for as long as it helps you stay focused even when the going gets tough.

- Strive to be good, not perfect

Intermittent fasting need neither be too academic nor too precise. Although faithfully adhering to the basics of your chosen fasting method is recommended, you need not panic upon knowing that you have somehow deviated from the routine. For example, there is no reason for you to freak out when you suddenly realize that you just ate a candy bar during your scheduled fasted period. Worry not for minor slips such as these won't hinder your progress for as long as you do your best to stick to the program and strive to avoid committing these mistakes again.

- Remember that there is no one-size-fits-all solution

The different intermittent fasting methods discussed in this book will yield different results for different people. In other words, you shouldn't force yourself to adapt to a specific method simply because someone you know is enjoying outstanding results doing that exact same thing. Your chosen fasting method will not work if you're going to force yourself to follow it. You should instead opt for a method that is sustainable for the long term, which will in turn make your life easier while giving you visible benefits.

- Know when to stop

Intermittent fasting is a way for you to attain better health through weight loss, not something that will put you in worse shape than before. Over time, if you find that the long periods of fasting are doing you more harm than good (i.e. stress, fatigue, etc.), don't push yourself any further. Talk with your doctor again to see if intermittent fasting really is for you or if there are other more viable weight loss methods available.

Conclusion

Thank you again for downloading this book!

I hope this book was able to teach you enough information about intermittent fasting as well as its benefits and how easy it really is to incorporate into your schedule. This is to encourage you to start practicing it to give your body the "rewiring" it needs to be able to more efficiently convert into energy the food you eat and ultimately limit the amount of unhealthy sugars and fats being stored within you.

Religiously following the structured eating plans and making better food choices can help you achieve weight loss. It will be challenging at first but you'll eventually realize that you aren't really depriving yourself of the things you need to live a happier and healthier life. Of course, you still need to talk with your doctor about your plans to determine which fasting method is most feasible for you.

The next step is to take what you have learned from this book and apply it in your weight loss efforts. May you enjoy success in your endeavors and encourage others to strive for the same!

Finally, if you enjoyed this book, then I'd like to ask you for a favor. I would really appreciate it if you could leave a review for this book on Amazon as this really helps smaller authors like me get in the limelight.

Thank you and good luck!